OTHER BOOKS BY THE AUTHOR

The Normal Child, 9th edition, 1987
Churchill Livingstone, Edinburgh
Translated into Greek, Spanish, Japanese, French,
Farsi and Italian

*The Development of the Infant and Young Child,
Normal and Abnormal*, 9th edition, 1987
Churchill Livingstone, Edinburgh
Translated into Japanese, French, Polish, Italian and
Spanish

*Lessons from Childhood: Some Aspects of the
Early Life of Unusual Men and Women*
with C. M. Illingworth, 1968
Churchill Livingstone, Edinburgh
Translated into Japanese

*Babies and Young Children: Feeding, Management
and Care*
with C. M. Illingworth, 7th edition, 1984
Churchill Livingstone, Edinburgh
Translated into Polish

*Treatment of the Child at Home: A Guide for Family
Doctors*, 1971
Blackwell Scientific Publications, Oxford
Translated into Greek

Common Symptoms of Disease in Children
9th edition, 1988
Blackwell Scientific Publications, Oxford
Translated into Spanish, Greek, Italian, Portuguese,
Indonesian, German and Japanese

*The Child at School: A Paediatrician's Manual for
Teachers*, 1975
Blackwell Scientific Publications, Oxford
Translated into Italian

Your Child's Development in the First Five Years, 1981
Churchill Livingstone, Edinburgh
Translated into Spanish

Infections and Immunization of your Child, 1981
Churchill Livingstone, Edinburgh
Translated into Spanish

Basic Developmental Screening: 0–4 years

RONALD S. ILLINGWORTH

MD (Leeds), Hon MD (Sheffield), Hon DSc (Baghdad), Hon DSc (Leeds),
FRCP (London), DPH, DCH
Emeritus Professor of Child Health
The University of Sheffield
Formerly Paediatrician to the
Children's Hospital and Paediatrician to the
Jessop Hospital for Women
The United Sheffield Hospitals

FIFTH EDITION

OXFORD

BLACKWELL SCIENTIFIC PUBLICATIONS

LONDON EDINBURGH BOSTON

MELBOURNE PARIS BERLIN VIENNA

© 1973, 1977, 1982, 1988, 1990 by
Blackwell Scientific Publications
Editorial Offices:
Osney Mead, Oxford OX2 0EL
25 John Street, London WC1N 2BL
23 Ainslie Place, Edinburgh EH3 6AJ
3 Cambridge Center, Suite 208,
   Cambridge, Massachusetts 02142,
   USA
54 University Street, Carlton
   Victoria 3053, Australia

First published 1973
Second edition 1977
Italian translation 1977
Japanese translation 1977
Greek translation 1978
Third edition 1982
Greek translation 1984
Fourth edition 1988
Spanish translation 1988
Fifth edition 1990
Reprinted 1991

Photoset by Enset (Photosetting),
Midsomer Norton, Bath, Avon
and printed and bound
in Great Britain by
The Alden Press, Oxford

DISTRIBUTORS

Marston Book Services Ltd
PO Box 87
Oxford OX2 0DT
(*Orders*: Tel: 0865 791155
          Fax: 0865 791927
          Telex: 837515)

USA
Year Book Medical Publishers
200 North LaSalle Street
Chicago, Illinois 60601
(*Orders*: Tel: (312) 726-9733)

Canada
The C.V. Mosby Company
5240 Finch Avenue East,
Scarborough, Ontario
(*Orders*: Tel: (416) 298-1588)

Australia
Blackwell Scientific Publications
(Australia) Pty Ltd,
54 University Street
Carlton, Victoria 3053
(*Orders*: Tel: (03) 347-0300)

British Library
Cataloguing in Publication Data

Illingworth, Ronald S. (Ronald
Stanley) 1909
   Basic development screening: 0–4
   years
   5th ed.
   1. Children, to 4 years. Physical
   development. Screening
   I. Title

ISBN 0–632–02905–6

Contents

v

Preface

This booklet is intended to be used for screening only. It is not intended to provide an accurate score, and is not intended to be used for research purposes. It is intended to provide the busy clinic doctor, general practitioner or hospital doctor with a rapid means of eliminating anything but the mildest developmental or neurological abnormality—and of knowing when to seek the advice of an expert when in doubt.

It is written in the firm belief that many have made developmental assessment far too complicated, and that there is a need for a brief, simple, practical guide to developmental screening. For more detailed assessment and for the basis and theory of assessment I hope that the reader will refer to my book *The Development of the Infant and Young Child, Normal and Abnormal*, 9th ed (1987), Churchill Livingstone, Edinburgh.

In this booklet I have mentioned only those features of development which are relevant and essential for screening purposes. I have aimed at keeping them to a minimum.

I have given careful consideration to material which I regard as essential and that which I regard as non-essential. *I do not consider that the elicitation of signs other than those described in this book are of value in ordinary routine developmental screening.* In particular I regard the elicitation of numerous primitive reflexes to be of no known importance for routine screening. Some may be of value to the specialist, but with rare exceptions I am sceptical even of this.

This edition has been thoroughly checked, with much rewriting. It includes a new section, with 16 sketches, concerning the preterm baby. I have placed particular emphasis, based on many years of experience, on the important errors to avoid in developmental assessment, especially in cerebral palsy and other handicaps.

Why screen?

Normal parents want to know whether their child is developing normally or not, particularly if there has been a difficulty with the previous pregnancy or previous child's development. The doctor needs to assess development if there has been some prenatal, perinatal or postnatal risk factor, or if there is some feature such as unusual developmental, behaviour or appearance. He needs to assess the effects of obstetrical or perinatal management, of drugs taken in pregnancy, and of a difficult delivery. He has to allay parental anxieties, to give advice about risks of future pregnancies, to discuss special educational needs, to determine the need of special treatment, or to assess suitability for adoption. He may be required to help in medicolegal matters concerning a claim of brain damage.

To the doctor, developmental screening is part of the routine examination of any baby.

THE BASIS OF SCREENING

The basis of screening is the comparison of the baby's level of development with that of an average baby of the same chronological age: it follows that a thorough knowledge of the 'average' or 'normal' is essential.

The following are the main principles of developmental assessment:

1 A child's level of development is the end result of a wide variety of factors—prenatal, perinatal and postnatal. Prenatal factors include genetic conditions, the family pattern of development (e.g. late sphincter control), viral infections, placental problems (including hypertension, bleeding, intrauterine growth retardation) and drugs, including alcohol and smoking; perinatal factors include difficulties in delivery, especially those involving hypoxia;

postnatal factors include trauma, effect of drugs, infections (e.g. meningitis) and management.

2 Development depends mainly on maturation of the relevant part of the nervous system. Hence in infancy allowance must always be made for preterm delivery. The assessment is not just made on 'milestones'; one not only needs to know *whether* a particular skill has been acquired, but also the maturity shown.

3 The mentally subnormal child is retarded in all fields of development, except sometimes gross motor development (sitting and walking) and rarely sphincter control.

4 All clinical diagnoses, such as developmental assess-. ment, must be made on the basis of history, full physical examination (e.g. for handicap, for which allowance has to be made), and the interpretation of the whole. An adequate assessment cannot be made purely on objective psychological tests, which ignore the relevant history, physical examination and the vitally important unscorable or less easily scorable items—such as concentration, alertness, interest in surroundings, responsiveness, power of observation, play behaviour and memory.

5 All children are different—because of the wide variety of relevant factors—and it is therefore impossible to lay down the *range* of normality; all one can say is that the further away from the average he is, the less likely he is to be 'normal'. It is absurd to say that a child 'should' do this, that and the other by a certain age.

6 It is unwise to attempt to give a single figure as a score for a child's performance and to term it the IQ. A single figure could be interpreted as implying, wrongly, that all aspects of development are of equal importance. It is wiser merely to indicate how far he has developed in relation to his age ('Developmental Quotient', DQ). One must then recognize that this will be profoundly modified by his home, friends, neighbours, health, nutrition, personality and many other factors. I suggest that a good way to report one's findings would be as follows:

The overall performance of this 24-month-old child is that of an average 30-month-old, with some scatter in the

2

range of 27 to 36 months. His overall development is therefore above average.

7   In developmental assessment there is no place for a 'spot diagnosis'. One must never be misled by a baby's charm, ugly appearance, odd-shaped head, bad behaviour, small size, or physical handicap, in such a way that his overall ability is wrongly estimated.

8   In making the final assessment, one puts all the findings of the history, physical and developmental examination, and all the factors which may have affected or be affecting his development, into one's cerebral computer and reaches a conclusion—which may later be modified by follow-up examination.

9   The only way to learn about developmental assessment is to follow up all children who present doubtful or difficult problems.

The preterm baby

For a better understanding of normal development, I have added 16 sketches (by courtesy of Churchill Livingstone) to show some of the differences between a 28–30 week preterm baby, and a full-term one.

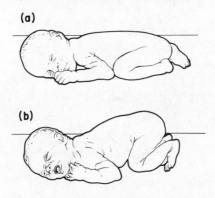

Fig. 1. *Prone. (a) Preterm: flat on couch, hips abducted.*
(b) Fullterm: pelvis high off couch, knees under trunk.

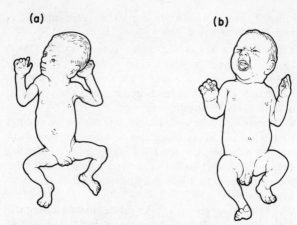

Fig. 2. *Supine. (a) Preterm: head rotated to side, hips abducted, so that lower limbs and knees are flat on couch. (b) Fullterm: head less rotated, hips not abducted, knees not on couch.*

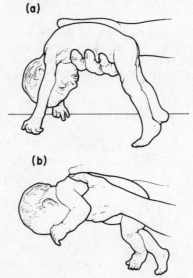

Fig. 3. *(a) Ventral suspension. Preterm: no extension of neck, arms and legs hang down, not flexed. (b) Fullterm: some extension at neck, elbows, knees flexed.*

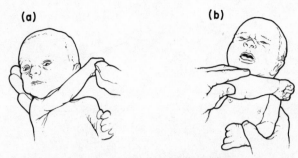

Fig. 4. *Scarf sign (arms passed in front of neck). (a) Preterm: hand reaches well beyond tip of shoulder. (b) Fullterm: hand reaches no further than tip of shoulder.*

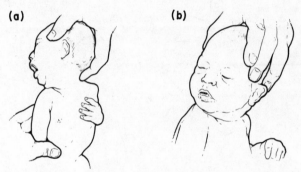

Fig. 5. *Head rotation. (a) Preterm: chin reaches beyond tip of shoulder. (b) Fullterm: chin will not reach beyond shoulder*

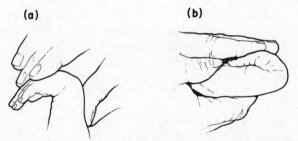

Fig. 6. *Wrist flexion. (a) Preterm "Window sign", flexion not nearly complete. (b) Fullterm: full flexion of wrist.*

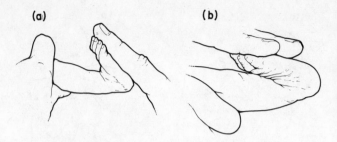

Fig. 7. *Dorsiflexion at ankle. (a) Preterm: dorsiflexion not nearly complete. (b) Fullterm: full dorsiflexion.*

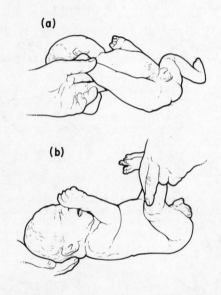

Fig. 8. *Hips fully flexed, flexion and extension of knee. (a) Preterm: full extension at knee. (b) Fullterm: incomplete extension at knee.*

Milestones of development
(after allowance for preterm delivery)

See Figs 9–46, pp. 8–19.

Most important milestones in italics.

Newborn   Prone—pelvis high, knees under abdomen.

2–4 weeks   Watches mother intently as she speaks to him.

1 month   Ventral suspension (held prone, hand under abdomen)—head up momentarily, elbows flexed, hips partly extended, knees flexed.

4–6 weeks   *Smiles at mother in response to overtures.*

6 weeks   *Ventral suspension—head held up momentarily in same plane as rest of body. Some extension of hips and flexion of knees and elbows. Prone—pelvis largely flat, hips mostly extended.*
(But when sleeping the baby lies with pelvis high, knees under abdomen, like a newborn baby.)
Pull to sit from the supine—much head lag, but not complete; hands often open.
Supine—follows object 90 cm away over angle of 90°.

2 months   Ventral suspension—maintains head in same plane as rest of body.
Hands largely open.
Prone—chin off couch. Plane of face 45° to couch.
Smiles and vocalizes when talked to.
Eyes—follow moving person.

continues on p. 20

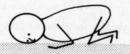

Fig. 9. *Newborn: prone—pelvis high, knees under abdomen.*

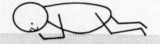

Fig. 10. *6 weeks: prone—pelvis flat, hips extended.*

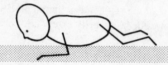

Fig. 11. *6 weeks: prone—chin intermittently lifted off couch.*

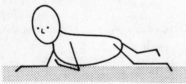

Fig. 12. *3 months: prone—weight on forearms, chest well off couch.*

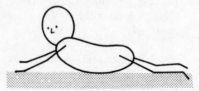

Fig. 13. *6 months: prone—weight on hands, arms extended.*

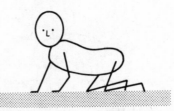

Fig. 14. *10 months: creep position—hands and knees.*

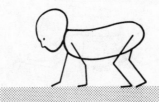

Fig. 15. *1 year: walking like a bear, on soles of feet and hands.*

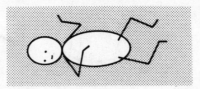

Fig. 16. *Newborn: supine, flexed position.*

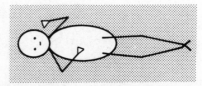

Fig. 17. *Newborn spastic: lower limbs extended.*

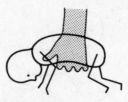

Fig. 18. *Newborn: ventral suspension—head held up a little, elbows flexed, hips partly extended.*

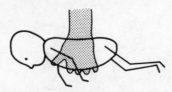

Fig. 19. *6 weeks: ventral suspension—head held up momentarily in same plane as rest of body. Hips extended.*

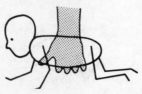

Fig. 20. *10 weeks: ventral suspension—head held up well beyond plane of rest of body.*

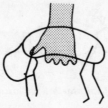

Fig. 21. *2 months: abnormal baby in ventral suspension—arms and legs hang down.*

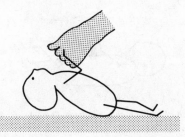

Fig. 22. *Newborn: pulled to sit—almost complete head lag.*

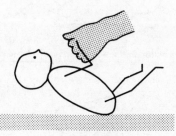

Fig. 23. *2 months: pulled to sit—less head lag.*

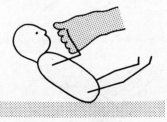

Fig. 24. *4 months: pulled to sit—no head lag.*

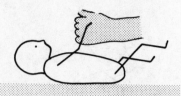

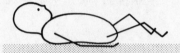

Fig. 25. *5 months: when about to be pulled up, lifts head.*

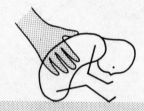

Fig. 26. *6 months: supine—spontaneously elevates head.*

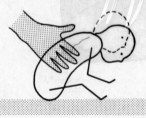

Fig. 27. *Newborn: held sitting—fully rounded back.*

Fig. 28. *1 month: held sitting—lifts head up intermittently.*

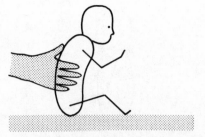

Fig. 29. *2 months: held sitting—back straightening; head up.*

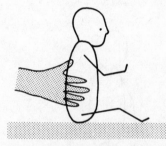

Fig. 30. *4 months: held sitting—head well up, steady, back nearly straight.*

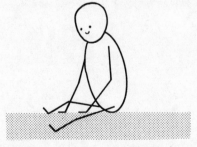

Fig. 31. *6 months: sits with hands forward for support.*

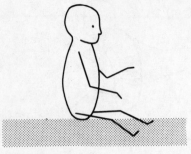

Fig. 32. *8 months: sitting steadily, no support.*

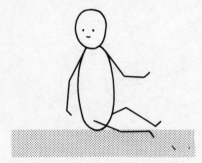

Fig. 33. *11 months: sits and pivots.*

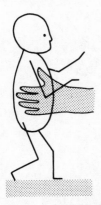
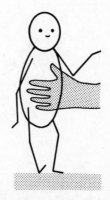

Fig. 34. *3 months: held standing—sags at knees and hips.*

Fig. 35. *6 months: held standing—bears full weight.*

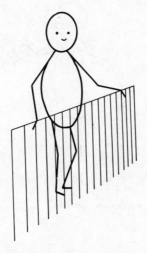

Fig. 36. *9 months: stands—holding on to playpen.*

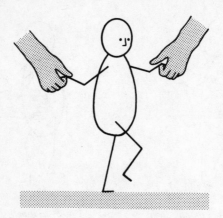

Fig. 37. *11 months: walks—2 hands held.*

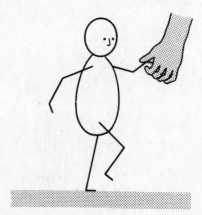

Fig. 38. *1 year: walks—one hand held.*

16

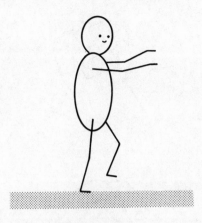

Fig. 39. *13 months: walks—no support.*

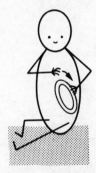

Fig. 40. *6 months: transfers from one hand to another.*

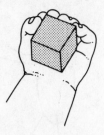

Fig. 41. *6 months: palmar grasp of cube.*

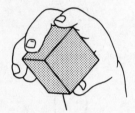

Fig. 42. *8 months: grasp, intermediate.*

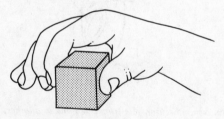

Fig. 43. *1 year: mature grasp of cube.*

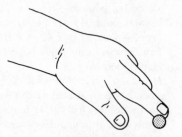

Fig. 44. *9–10 months: index finger approach to object.*

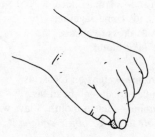

Fig. 45. *9–10 months: finger–thumb apposition—pellet picked up between tip of forefinger and tip of thumb.*

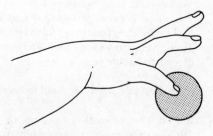

Fig. 46. *6 months (or older): spastic approach to object—splaying out of hand.*

19

3 months	Ventral suspension—holds head up long time beyond plane of rest of body.
	Prone—plane of face 45°–90° from couch.
	Pulled to sit—only slight head lag.
	Hands loosely open.
	Holds rattle placed in hand.
	Vocalizes a great deal when talked to.
	Follows object for 180° (lying supine).
	Turns head to sound (3–4 months) on a level with the ear.
4 months	Prone—plane of face at 90° to couch.
	Hands come together.
	Pulls dress over face.
	Laughs aloud.
5 months	Prone—weight on forearms.
	Pulled to sit—no head lag.
	Supine—feet to mouth. Plays with toes.
	Able to go for object and get it.
6 months	Prone—weight on hands, extended arms.
	Pulled to sit—no head lag.
	Supine—lifts head spontaneously.
	Sits on floor, hands forward for support.
	Held in standing position—full weight on legs.
	Rolls, prone to supine, completely over.
	Begins to imitate (e.g. a cough).
	Chews.
	Transfers cube from one hand to another.
7 months	*Sits on floor for seconds, no support.*
	Rolls, supine to prone, completely over.
	Held standing—bounces.
	Feeds self with biscuit.
	Attracts attention by cough or other method.
	Attracts head to sound below level of ear.

| 8 months | Sits unsupported. Leans forward to reach objects. |
| | Turns head to sound above level of ear. |

| 9 months | Stands, holding on. Pulls to stand or sitting position. |
| | *Crawls on abdomen.* |

| 9–10 months | *Index finger approach.* |
| | *Finger-thumb apposition*—picks pellet between tip of thumb and tip of forefinger. |

10 months	*Creeps, hands and knees, abdomen off couch.*
	Can change from sitting to prone and back.
	Pulls self to sitting position.
	Waves bye.
	Plays pat-a-cake.
	Helps to dress—holding arm out for coat, foot for shoe, or transferring object from one hand to another for sleeve.

11 months	*Offers object to mother, but will not release it.*
	One word with meaning.
	Sitting—pivots round without overbalancing.
	Walks, holding on to furniture; walks, 2 hands held.

1 year	2–3 words with meaning.
	Prone—walks on hands and feet like bear.
	Walks, one hand held.
	Casting objects, one after another, begins.
	Gives brick to mother.

13 months	*Walks, no support.*
	Mouthing of objects largely stopped.
	Slobbering largely stopped.

| 15 months | Creeps up stairs. Kneels. |
| | Takes off shoes. |

Feeds self, picking up an ordinary cup,
drinking, putting it down.
Imitation of mother in domestic work
('domestic mimicry').
Jargon.
Cubes—tower of 2.

18 months   *No more casting.*
Gets up and down stairs, holding rail.
Jumps, both feet.
Seats self in chair.
Toilet control—tells mother that he wants
potty. Largely dry by day.
Throws ball without falling.
Takes off gloves, socks, unzips.
Manages spoon well.
Points to 3 parts of body on request.
Book—turns pages, 2 or 3 at a time.
Points to some objects, on request.
Cubes—tower of 3-4.
Pencil and paper—imitates stroke (examiner
gets child to watch stroke being made and asks
child to do the same). Picture card—identifies
one. (Where is the?)

21–24   *Spontaneously joins 2 or 3 words together to*
months   *make sentence.*

2 years   Picks up object from floor without falling.
Runs.
Kicks ball without overbalancing.
Turns door knob.
Cubes—tower of 6 or 7.
Puts on shoes, socks, pants; takes off shoes,
socks.
Points to 4 parts of body on request.
Pencil—imitates vertical and circular strokes.
Book—turns pages singly.
Mainly dry at night.

	Climbs stairs, 2 feet per step. Cubes—imitates train but forgets chimney. Picture card—identifies 5 (Where is the?). Names 3 (What is this?).
2½ years	Knows full name, sex. Cubes—tower of 8. Imitates train with chimney. Picture card—identifies 7, names 5. Pencil and paper—imitates vertical and horizontal strokes. Digits (say after me, e.g. 825), 3 trials (different figures in each trial). Two in one of 3 trials. Coloured forms—places one correctly.
3 years	Dresses and undresses fully, except shoe laces. Cubes—tower of 9. Imitates bridge. Pencil and paper—imitates cross (i.e. watches examiner make one). Pencil and paper—copies circle (i.e. copies previously prepared circle). Picture card—names 8. Digits—3 in one of 3 trials. Coloured forms—3 correct. Uncoloured forms—4 correct.
3½ years	Cubes—tower of 10. Copies bridge (i.e. examiner made bridge out of sight of child). Picture card—names 10. Digits—3 correct in 2 of 3 trials. Uncoloured forms—6.
4 years	Cubes—imitates gate. Pencil and paper—copies train. Digits—3 in 3 of 3 trials. Coloured forms—all correct. Uncoloured forms—8.

Age for screening

The easiest ages at which to screen babies after the newborn examination are 6 weeks, 6 months and 10 months. This is because there are readily assessable features of development at those ages. The most difficult age at which to screen after the newborn period is 3 to 4 months, and I prefer not to assess a baby at 8 months. From the age of 1 to about 3 it is particularly difficult, because children are coy, shy and in the phase of negativism.

General history

The history must include:

Birth weight and duration of gestation.

Prenatal and perinatal risk factors—see p. 1.

Postnatal—development (e.g. age of beginning to smile, etc.), sucking or swallowing difficulties, undue drowsiness, irritability, crying, illness, emotional deprivation, social factors.

The previous development of the baby has to be determined. In order to assess the previous rate of development one needs to know whether there are signs that a child who has had a bad start is showing accelerated development (and may therefore catch up to the normal), slowing of development (as in degenerative diseases of the nervous system) or signs of deterioration in performance. One must know whether there has been any illness or other factor such as emotional deprivation which may have retarded his development. The 'risk' factors will be named in the relevant sections to follow.

If there is delay in development, a history of the familial

pattern of development is important. For instance, if the child is late in sitting and walking, and is normal in other aspects of development, one may find that the father or ·mother was similarly late in motor development.

Developmental history

It is essential that the doctor and mother should each understand what the other means and says. One assesses the mother's understanding, memory and veracity as she replies, and when in doubt comes back and asks the same question in a different way. The questions to be asked depend on the age of the child: it would not be profitable to ask the mother of a 5-year-old, who was one of 10 children, when he began to smile. It is not enough to ask *whether* he shows a particular skill. One needs to know *when* he began to show it.

The developmental history is a good comparative check on one's own objective findings. The following are suggested questions when the child is of a relevant age (corrected for prematurity):

1 Does he smile at you when you talk to him? I mean only when you talk to him. When did he begin? (Av. 4–6 weeks.) Some mothers have the extraordinary idea that pain from wind makes babies smile. They may interpret any facial movement in sleep as a smile: or else they stroke the lips or face and interpret a facial movement as a smile. The doctor is interested only in the smile in response to social overture.

2 Does he make little cooing noises as well as smile when you talk to him? When did he begin? (Av. a week or 2 after smiling begins.) Later, when doubtful about possible backwardness, one asks, 'Does he smile much?' A backward child at 6 months may smile only occasionally.

3 Will he hold a rattle if you put it in the hand? How long? When did he begin? (Av. 3–4 months.)

4 Does he turn his head when he hears noises? When did he begin? (Av. 3–4 months.)

5 Will he reach out for a toy and get it without it being put into the hand? When did he begin? (Av. 5 months.) If one has difficulty in eliciting the response with the cube, ask 'Would he be able to get hold of this without it being put into the hand?'

6 Have you seen him take a toy from one hand into the other? When did he begin? (Av. 6 months.)

7 Can he chew yet? I do not mean 'suck'. Does he make chewing movements with the jaw? Can he manage to eat a biscuit? When did he begin? (Av. 6–7 months.) (This is nothing to do with teething.)

8 Can he sit on the floor without support? When did he begin to sit for a few seconds on the floor without help? (Av., with hands forward for support—6 months; with no support, for seconds—7 months.) (*Note*. This is very different from sitting in the pram, with support round the buttocks, etc.)

9 Does he copy you in anything that you do? If the mother says 'yes', ask her what he does. He may imitate a noise, razzing or a cough, or putting the tongue out. When did he begin? (Av. 6–7 months.)

10 Will he stand, holding on to the furniture? When did he begin? (Av. 8 months.)

11 Will he pull himself up to the standing position at the side of the furniture? When did he begin? (Av. 9 months.)

12 Does he crawl (on his tummy) (av. 9 months) or creep (hands and knees)? (Av. 10 months.) When did he begin?

13 Does he walk, holding on to the furniture ('cruise')? When did he begin? (Av. 10 months.)

14 Will he wave bye-bye? When did he begin? (Av. 9 months.)

15 Will he play pat-a-cake (clap hands)? When did he begin? (Av. 9 months.)

16 Does he say any words with meaning? (Av. 10–11 months.) If the mother claims that he says 'dada' one asks,

'Does he really mean daddy? Is it when daddy is not there or only when he is there?'

17 Does he help you to dress him? If the answer is 'yes', ask what he does. One means that he holds his arm out for a coat, foot out for a shoe, or passes an object from one hand into the other in order to put his arm into a sleeve. When did he begin? (Av. 10 months.)

18 Can he manage an ordinary cup—to pick it up, drink from it and put it down—without you helping him? When did he begin? (Av. 15 months.) Does he feed himself fully without help? (Av. 15–18 months.)

19 Can he dress himself or undress himself at all? What can he get on or off? When did he begin? (Av., shoes and socks off at 15 months; takes off gloves, socks, unzips at 18 months; puts on shoes, socks, pants at 2 years.)

20 Does he tell you when he wants to use the potty? When did he begin? (Av. 18 months.) Is he usually dry by day? (Av. 24 months.) By night? (Av. 2–3 years.)

21 Does he copy you doing things about the house—brushing, sweeping, washing up? (Domestic mimicry.) When did he begin? (Av. 15 months.)

22 Does he join 2 or 3 words together (not just imitating you)? When did he begin? (Av. 21–24 months.)

If in doubt about a child's hearing, ask 'Will he come from another room if called—without his seeing you call him?'

If in doubt about his being backward in speech—ask 'Does he understand what you say to him? Could he point out objects in pictures if you ask him?' (Understanding of words always precedes the ability to articulate them.)

If in doubt about his being backward, and if he has older siblings at school, ask, 'How does he compare with his brother/sister, apart from his speech? (if he is late in talking). What about his general understanding, his intelligence? Then ask, 'Is his brother/sister doing well at school?' (in case he is also backward).

Equipment

The equipment needed for the physical examination is a stethoscope, patellar hammer (a small one preferably with a triangular piece of rubber at the tapping end), a non-stretch tape-measure (for many tape-measures stretch and become inaccurate), a head circumference chart, and a weight and height chart (with centiles). Scales for weighing should be checked for accuracy at intervals.

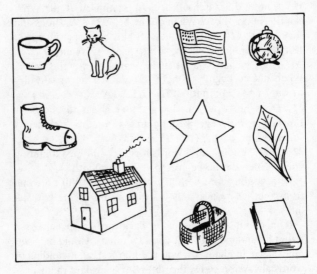

Fig. 47. *Two 'picture cards' (30×22.5 cm).*

The essential equipment for development screening is 10 one inch cubes (only 2 or 3 are needed in the first year), a fairly blunt-ended pencil and paper, a picture card (Fig. 47), and coloured and uncoloured cut-out shapes to fit into corresponding places on the card (Figs 48–49). Figure 50 shows the tower, train, bridge, gate and steps constructed from the cubes.

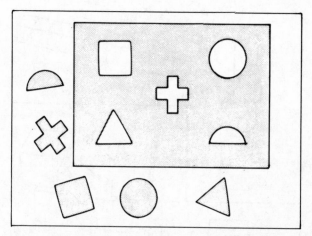

Fig. 48. *Red 'coloured forms', cut out of cardboard. (Whole card measures 30×22.5 cm; shapes to correspond, e.g. the square measures 5×5 cm.)*

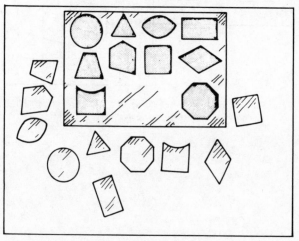

Fig. 49. *'Uncoloured forms'. (Whole card measures 30×22.5 cm; shapes to correspond, e.g. the square measures 5×5 cm.)*

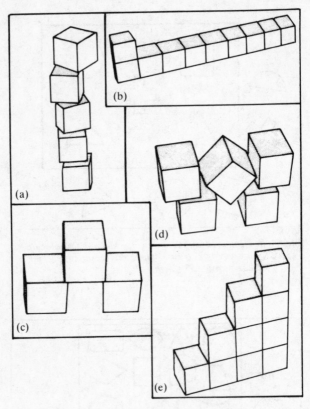

Fig. 50. One inch cubes. (a) Tower of 5 cubes; (b) train with chimney; (c) bridge; (d) gate; (e) steps.

Physical and developmental examination

The physical and developmental examination must include examination for congenital abnormalities, such as limb deformities, cleft palate, congenital heart diesease, visual or auditory defects because a child with any major congenital abnormality is more liable than others to be mentally

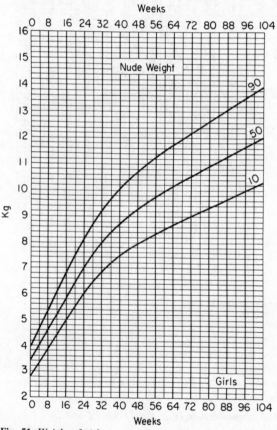

Fig. 51. *Weight of girls.*

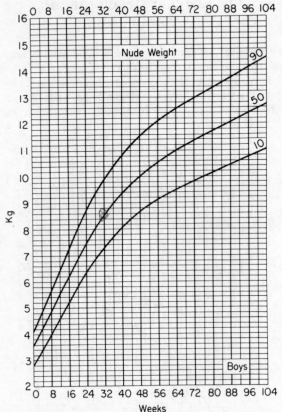

Fig. 52. *Weight of boys.*

below average, and because allowance must be made for them in the assessment. It will include examination for subluxation or dislocation of the hip (p. 58). It must include the maximum head circumference in relation to the baby's weight.

Head circumference (Fig. 53, Tables 1a and 2)

The maximum head circumference must be determined in

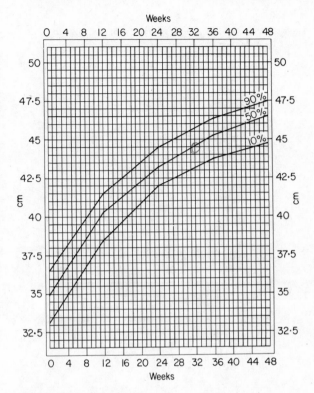

Fig. 53. *Head circumference.*

all babies as a routine because the head size depends on the growth of the cranial contents. If the brain does not grow normally the head circumference is likely to be small and so suggests a brain defect; but a normal head circumference does not always eliminate a defect of the brain. If mental subnormality develops after about 12 months (e.g. as a result of trauma or meningitis), the head will not be significantly small, because most of the brain's growth has occurred by that age.

An unusually large head may indicate hydrocephalus or other disease. In all cases the head circumference must be related to the baby's weight, for a big baby is likely to

Table 1a. *Head circumference in relation to birth weight.* (After Usher R. & McLean F. (1969) *J. Pediatr.* **74,** 901.)

Birth weight (g)	Head circumference (cm)
1000	24.5
1200	26.2
1400	27.7
1600	29.0
1800	30.1
2000	31.0
2200	31.8
2400	32.5
2600	33.1
2800	33.6
3000	34.1
3200	34.5
3400	34.9
3600	35.2
3800	35.5
4000	35.8

Table 1b. *Mean birth weight at different gestation periods.*

Duration of gestation (weeks)	Mean birth weight (g)
26	933
28	1113
30	1373
32	1727
34	2113
36	2589
38	3133
40	3480

have a bigger head than a small baby, and a small baby a smaller head than a big baby.

An incorrect diagnosis of hydrocephalus can be made by failing to relate a rapid increase in head size on the centile chart to the correspondingly rapid increase in the weight gain. When in doubt the head circumference and the weight should be plotted on the centile charts: they should more or less correspond in their placing—though

Screening at 18 months

As before, if not already taken. In addition ask:

How many words he says with meaning.

Whether he is joining any words together, other than in imitation, and when he began.

When he walked without help.

When he was able to feed himself fully, managing an ordinary cup, picking it up, drinking and putting it down without help.

How much he can dress and undress himself.

Whether he tells the mother that he wants the potty, when he began, and when he was usually dry—by day or by night.

When he began domestic mimicry.

If he seems backward, ask how long he will play with one toy. (Distinguish the obsessional play of a retarded child with one toy.)

EXAMINATION

Observe facial expression, alertness, responsiveness, interest in surroundings, skull size and shape, jargon, speech.

Observe mouthing, slobbering, casting—all probably abnormal at this age.

Observe the eyes—squint, nystagmus, opacity.

Test the hearing.

Only test for the index finger approach and finger-thumb apposition if he is backward.

Offer 6 bricks: show him how to build a tower.

Ask him to point to parts of the body, or his shoe, or to fetch a ball.

Test for distant vision.

Take him from his mother, after removing the nappy.

Test hip abduction, muscle tone, knee jerks, plantar responses.

Examine the heart, palpate the abdomen and testes.

Observe his gait as he walks.
Measure the head circumference, as before.

Screening at 2 years

HISTORY REQUIRED

As before, if not already taken; exclude developmental history prior to 6 months.
In addition the age of onset of:
  Joining words together.
  Toilet training: dryness day and night.
  Ability to dress self: how much he can do.
  Ability to feed self.

EXAMINATION

As 18-month child.
If speech is delayed, ask whether he understands everything said to him, whether he can hear and whether he will come from another room if called without seeing the mother call him.
Offer 6 cubes. Make a train of 5 with a chimney and ask him to do the same: he is unlikely to add the chimney.
Observe mouthing, slobbering or casting (all abnormal at this age).
Ask him to point to parts of the body.

Interpretation

1 Preterm delivery

Allowance *must* be made. For example, when assessing a 6-month-old baby, who was born 2 months prematurely, one compares him not with an average 6-month baby, but with a 4-month-old baby. It could be argued that environmental factors after birth could affect the validity of full allowance for prematurity.

2 Optimum performance

One has to be satisfied that the child's performance was probably the best of which he was capable. One must not assess a baby when he is tired, hungry, bored or under the influence of drugs.

When in doubt, one checks one's objective findings with his mother's account of his skills or milestones.

3 Previous rate of development

This is assessed on the basis of the mother's account. It helps one to consider whether his development is steady, accelerating (as in the occasional 'slow starter') or slowing.

4 Minimum developmental level

It is often important to note an infant's minimum developmental level. For instance, a baby who spontaneously lifts his head from the supine cannot be less than the 6-month level of motor development. A baby who transfers an object from one hand to another cannot be less than the 6-month level of manipulation: if he shows the index finger approach to an object he cannot be less than the 9–10 month level of manipulation, and because of the importance of this aspect of development he can hardly be less than the 10-month level of intellectual development.

5 Relative importance of different fields of development

Some aspects of development are far more important for overall assessment than others. For instance, gross motor development (sitting and walking) are the least important (but most easily scored): some mentally subnormal infants sit and walk at the average age. Advanced motor development certainly does not mean high intelligence. Manipulative development, the use of the hands, especially the index finger approach and the finger tip and thumb tip grasp are much more important. If the index finger approach and finger-tip–thumb apposition are seen at the average age (9 to 10 months) mental subnormality can be virtually excluded.

45

Much the most important features for assessment are unscorable: they are the child's alertness, responsiveness, rapidity of response, concentration, imitation, the quality of his vocalization. Teething is of no importance in assessment.

It follows that it is totally wrong to put a score on say 5 different aspects of development, add the scores up, divide by 5, and conclude that this denotes his overall developmental level.

6 Allowance for factors affecting development

These include prematurity and familial pattern, (e.g. family age of motor development, speech, sphincter control, and later reading). They must include allowance for handicaps, including visual, auditory and motor difficulties, and adverse social or management factors, such as emotional deprivation or malnutrition. One may have to exclude tests which are affected by a particular handicap—such as weight bearing if the child has a meningomyelocele, or speech if he is deaf.

7 Significance of risk factors

Risk factors are important, but their importance must not be exaggerated. For instance, a mentally subnormal mother may have a mentally normal child. If after assessment the child is normal, the risk factors (unless they concern degenerative diseases of the nervous system or serious psychoses) are usually ignored, but if there are doubtful aspects of development, the risk factor increases the likelihood that all is not well. For instance, if a child had a very low birth weight, he is at risk of cerebral palsy, but if on examination there is delayed motor development (after allowance for preterm delivery), then there is a greater likelihood that he has cerebral palsy (or mental subnormality). Any major congenital abnormality is a risk factor, increasing the possibility that there is associated mental subnormality.

8 Variations in certain fields of development (after allowing for prematurity)

SMILING

I have seen children smiling in response by 2 or 3 days after birth. I would be concerned if smiling had not begun by 8 weeks if full-term.

Late smiling   Lack of stimulation by parents.

                      Mental subnormality.

                      Blindness.

                      Autism.

                      Mobius syndrome.

MOTOR DEVELOPMENT

I have seen normal children sitting without support by 5 months, or not till 12 months, and normal children walking without support by 7 months, or not till 4 years.

Late sitting   Familial.
and walking   Mental subnormality.

                      Hypotonia or hypertonia (cerebral palsy).

                      Emotional deprivation.

                      Environmental factors; the mother keeping
                         the child off his feet.

                      Muscular dystrophy.

                      Blindness.

Late walking is unlikely to be due to dislocated hip or obesity.

Some babies miss the stage of creeping.

SPEECH

I have seen normal children join words together by 10 months, or not till 5 years of age.

Understanding of speech long precedes ability to articulate, and is far more important for assessment.

Late speech   Familial.

                      Environmental—no one talking to the child.

                      Multiple pregnancy.

                      Mental subnormality.

                      Deafness.

Autism.

Unexplained.

Late speech is *not* due to laziness, jealousy, or everything being done for the child, or tongue tie.

SPHINCTER CONTROL

I have seen normal children with full control by 15 months, or not until 10 years or later.

Late control : causes Familial feature.

Delayed maturation of relevant part of the nervous system.

Mismanagement.

Psychological stress, especially at the time control is usually acquired.

Organic disease—mental retardation, urinary tract infection, development of polyuria at the time control is usually acquired, spina bifida, absent sacral segments, diastematomyelia, urethral valves (male) or ectopic ureter (female) causing dribbling incontinence.

Delay is *not* purely psychological, but psychological factors may be superimposed on other causes.

When should expert advice be sought?

1 Significant lateness in any field of development.

2 Combination of significant risk factors with doubtful development, or failure to thrive, especially if there is defective physical growth or emotional deprivation.

3 Suspected visual or auditory defect, cerebral palsy or hip dislocation.

4 A boy who has not walked by 18 months should have a laboratory test to exclude muscular dystrophy

Avoid causing worry

One should avoid, as far as possible, raising any doubt in the mind of the mother, until one decides that the child must be seen by a specialist. The slightest suggestion that a child may be spastic, retarded or hydrocephalic will cause the greatest anxiety. Even the doctor's facial expression may reveal to the mother the fact that he is doubtful about features of the examination. But the mother has to be told if he suspects a condition for which treatment would be required—or if he is assessing a baby for adoption.

A false positive diagnosis of an abnormality, such as hydrocephalus, mental subnormality or cerebral palsy, when the child is in fact normal, will cause great distress. A false negative diagnosis (i.e. saying that the child is normal when he is not) will cause much anger—and may have medicolegal consequences.

What we can and cannot do in developmental assessment

We can diagnose:
(i)   Moderate or severe cases of mental subnormality, cerebral palsy and other neurological defects, hearing or visual defects.
(ii) Subluxation of the hip.
We cannot:
(i)   Draw the line between normal and abnormal—and therefore state the range of normal.
(ii) Reliably diagnose the mildest mental subnormality or mildest cerebral palsy in early infancy.
(iii) Reliably assess a preterm baby until 4 to 6 weeks after he has reached the equivalent of full term.
(iv) Reliably diagnose mental superiority in early infancy.

(v) Predict in early infancy the possible disappearance of abnormal neurological signs.

(vi) Prove that a child's mental subnormality or cerebral palsy is due to birth injury.

(vii) Predict the reversibility of damage by emotional deprivation or severely adverse socioeconomic factors.

Mistakes to avoid

1 Failure to take a full history, including familial features.

2 Failure to base opinion on examination of the child as a whole, consideration of handicap, illnesses, malnutrition, anaemia.

3 Failure to recognize that at the time of testing the child was tired, hungry or ill, so that his performance was deceptively poor.

4 Diagnosis based on single items, instead of on a combination of items. Diagnosis based on appearance or behaviour only.

5 Failure to recognize great normal variations in all fields of development, especially those related to familial traits, or the overall course of development, the slow starter, unexpected improvement especially after the newborn period or an illness.

6 Failure to consider all factors which may have affected his development or may do so in the future—illnesses, drugs, environment, deterioration.

7 Failure to remember that some retarding factors may not appear till the child is much older—clumsiness, visuospatial difficulties, learning disorders, the effect of illness, drugs or environment.

Mental subnormality

Risk factors, which increase the likelihood that a child may be mentally retarded, are mainly:

Prenatal   Low birth weight, in relation to the duration of gestation. Extreme prematurity.

Family history of mental subnormality.
Virus infections in early pregnancy.
Pelvic irradiation.

Natal   Severe perinatal hypoxia.
Neonatal convulsions, especially if due to hypoglycaemia.
Hyperbilirubinaemia.

Postnatal   Hypoglycaemic fits.
Pyogenic meningitis.
Lead poisoning.
Emotional deprivation, malnutrition.
Severe head injury.

The mentally subnormal infant is late in all aspects of development, except occasionally in gross motor development (sitting and walking): he is relatively more advanced in sitting and walking than in other fields unless there is associated cerebral palsy, in which case he will be more retarded in motor development than in other fields. He is relatively more retarded in responsiveness, alertness and interest in surroundings, and later in speech, than in other fields. Mental subnormality can never be diagnosed on the basis of retardation in single fields of development, but only on a combination of signs and symptoms.

There is usually a small head circumference in relation to the weight: but there may be hydrocephalus.

There are often other congenital anomalies (such as congenital heart disease, cleft palate, syndactyly).

As he is late in all fields of development, with the occasional exceptions noted, the following are some of the developmental features of the mentally subnormal infant:

1 In the newborn period, he is more likely to have sucking, swallowing and feeding difficulties.

2 He sleeps more than most normal babies. Mothers often describe their backward babies as being 'so good, not a bit of trouble'.

3 He is late in:

Smiling in response to his mother, and subsequently in vocalizing.

Following with his eyes and in turning his head to sound. His response is slow.

Reaching out for objects and getting them.

Learning to chew.

Imitating, e.g. a cough, pat-a-cake, waving bye-bye.

Helping his mother to dress him.

Ceasing to take toys and other objects to the mouth.

Later (after the 1st birthday) ceasing to 'cast' (throw) one object after another onto the floor (normally stopped after about 15 months).

4 *He shows poor interest in his surroundings, less alertness and responsiveness than normal babies. He is too easily distracted so that he does not concentrate, e.g. on trying to reach an object.*

Mental deterioration

The following are the main causes of either slowing in development or mental deterioration:

Malnutrition in infancy.

Emotional deprivation. Child abuse.

Hyperbilirubinaemia, neonatal.

Metabolic diseases—phenylketonuria, other abnormal amino-acidurias, lipoidoses, mucopolysaccharidoses.

Hypothyroidism.

Hypoglycaemia.

Hypernatraemia.
Lead poisoning.
Epilepsy, and overdose of anticonvulsant drugs.
Degenerative diseases of the nervous system.
Meningitis.
Cerebral vascular accidents.
Severe head injury.
Psychoses.
Hypoxia.
Children with Down's syndrome are developmentally more advanced in the early weeks. Their development slows down in the 2nd half of the 1st year.

Cerebral palsy
(See Figs 17, 21, 46)

There are several degrees of severity of cerebral palsy. The mildest forms cannot be diagnosed in infancy, but there should be no difficulty in diagnosing the moderate or severe forms in early infancy, especially those of the spastic variety.

History
Certain factors increase the risk that a child will have cerebral palsy. They are mainly:

Prenatal factors—low birth weight, especially extreme prematurity, intrauterine growth retardation, viral infection in pregnancy.

Relative infertility (long period before conception, repeated miscarriages, etc.).

Familiy history of cerebral palsy.

Multiple pregnancy.

Mental subnormality.

Severe prenatal or perinatal hypoxia.

Neonatal hyperbilirubinaemia.

Certain other features of the history may be helpful.

There may be sucking and swallowing difficulties in the newborn period. A mother may notice that her baby feels stiff, or that one arm and leg is stiff, or that one hand is kept closed (spastic hemiplegia) when the other is open, or that the kick is asymmetrical, or that on creeping one leg trails behind.

1 Spastic form

The following are the principal signs:

1 A moderately or severely spastic infant lies relatively immobile.

2 The hands are likely to be kept tightly closed, whereas a normal baby after 2 or 3 months keeps the hands predominantly open.

3 The head circumference is commonly small in relation to the weight, on account of the associated mental subnormality, and for the same reason the child is commonly backward in all aspects of development; there may be diminished alertness.

4 There is likely to be defective motor development in ventral suspension and in the prone position, with excessive head lag when he is pulled from the supine to the sitting position; but *sometimes there is excessive extensor tone, so that the child seems to have good head control in ventral suspension and the prone position, but this contrasts with the excessive head lag when he is pulled to the sitting position.*

5 When he is being pulled up from the supine position one may feel resistance because of spasm of the erector spinae, glutei and hamstrings; with one's hand in the popliteal space one feels the spasm of the hamstrings and notes the flexion of the knees as he is pulled up (meaning that he does not sit with the legs forward flat on the couch); and *when placed sitting forward he repeatedly falls back.* He may tend to rise onto the feet.

6 The knee jerks are exaggerated and there may be a sustained ankle clonus. The plantar responses are extensor.

The signs will be:

1 Increased muscle tone in the affected limb. Exaggerated knee jerks. Perhaps ankle clonus. Extensor plantar response.

2 Excessive extensor tone—as no. 5 (p. 54).

3 Defective head control.

4 Often signs of mental subnormality and a head circumference which is small in relation to his weight.

5 In the case of hemiplegia, apart from the above, shortening of the affected limb (leg or arm—more easy to detect in the leg), and unless both limbs are warm as a result of being in a warm room, the affected limb will be cold as compared with the normal side. There may be asymmetry of movement (e.g. in kicking).

6 A spastic approach to an object. When an object such as the shining handle of a patellar hammer or a cube is offered to the child who is old enough and mature enough to reach out and get it, the spastic hand splays out in a characteristic way when reaching for it (Fig. 46).

The signs will be the same as in the 4–8 month period. After this age, a characteristic feature of the spastic child is the development of toe walking (p. 57).

2 Athetoid form

Athetosis may be genetic, or due to hyperbilirubinaemia (kernicterus) or severe hypoxia (prenatal or perinatal).

The signs of severe kernicterus appear between about the 6th and 10th day: the signs are stiffness, opisthotonos, rolling of the eyes, a high-pitched cry, drowsiness, food refusal, irritability and loss of the Moro reflex. There is often a characteristic posture in the lower arms, with pronation of the wrist.

After this period the signs are indefinite: they include hypertonia (but occasionally hypotonia), with delayed motor development, and perhaps a head circumference small in relation to the weight, with other signs of mental subnormality. In severe cases there may be rhythmical tongue thrusting. When the child is old enough and mature enough to reach out for objects, he will have an ataxic approach, different from the splaying out of the spastic hand. The awkward movements of the spastic hand may lead to the incorrect diagnosis of athetosis, or of cerebral palsy of mixed spastic and athetoid type. But the plantar responses in the athetoid child are flexor and the knee jerks are normal. It is easy to underestimate the intellectual ability of an athetoid.

Many other conditions are associated with involuntary movements, including spasmus nutans and torsion spasm (see Illingworth, R.S. (1988) *Common Symptoms of Disease in Children*, 9th edition, Blackwell Scientific Publications).

When he is older the child with kernicterus may have difficulty in vertical gaze, enamel hypoplasia in the deciduous teeth, high tone deafness and athetoid movements: but the abnormal movements are not likely to be detected until after the first year.

Snares in the diagnosis of cerebral palsy

1 There are wide normal variations in muscle tone, in briskness of tendon reflexes, and in gross motor development. Only experience can tell one what to regard as within normal limits.

2 Unusually brisk tendon jerks in the young baby, often with ankle clonus and increased tone, may disappear as the baby gets older. The longer the signs persist, the more likely they are to be significant.

3 In assessing tone, one can be misled by voluntary resistance to passive movement, joint disease, or by muscle contracture, as in the relatively immobile baby with spina bifida or severe hypotonia.

4 Hypotonia is often wrongly diagnosed in the early weeks of the spastic child, because of the poor head control

in pulling him to the sitting position, but there are signs of hypertonia elsewhere, as in limited hip abduction.

5 Excessive extensor tone is easily missed (p. 54).

6 Weakness of muscle, as in Erb's palsy, should not be confused with cerebral palsy, because of the hypertonia in the latter.

7 The diagnosis must never be made on individual signs, instead of a combination of signs. One would pay little attention to one sign, such as ankle clonus, unless there were other signs, such as a small head in relation to weight, or delayed motor development. The diagnosis of cerebral palsy can never be made on the basis of isolated motor delay.

8 Weakness or spasticity of the limbs may be due to a spinal cord lesion instead of a cerebral one. True spastic paraplegia is rare. Minimal upper limb involvement, which would mean spastic diplegia, not paraplegia, could be missed by inadequate examination. (In the same way, spastic monoplegia is extremely rare; careful examination will almost always show that another limb is involved, so that the correct diagnosis is spastic hemiplegia.)

9 Degenerative diseases of the nervous system, such as Friedreich's ataxia. In that condition the knee jerks are absent, the plantar responses are extensor, and there is likely to be pes cavus and Rombergism.

10 The mildest forms of cerebral palsy may not be found till around school age, when examination of a clumsy child, who has been blamed for bad writing or laziness, may reveal minimal signs of cerebral palsy.

11 *Toe walking* commonly causes a wrong diagnosis of cerebral palsy, in which it is a common feature. But it is often merely a habit when a baby is learning to walk: there will be no other signs of cerebral palsy, such as limited hip abduction, and observation shows that the child frequently puts his feet flat on the ground.

Congenital shortening of the Achilles tendon causes toe walking with limited ankle dorsiflexion. In spastic cerbral palsy, when the knee is flexed, the limited ankle dorsiflexion disappears, but it persists if there is shortening of the Achilles tendon.

Other causes of toe walking are unilateral dislocation of the hip, Duchenne muscular dystrophy, peroneal muscular atrophy, spinal tumour, dystonia musculorum deformans and infantile autism.

The hips

Risk factors
Factors which are associated with a special risk of subluxation of the hip include the following:
Family history of dislocated hip.
Geographical factors. The condition is more common in some areas (e.g. north Italy) than others.
Breech delivery, especially with extended legs.
Sternomastoid tumour (*congenital torticollis*).
Severe hypotonia.
Spasticity.
Bilateral talipes in a girl.
Arthrogryposis.
Intrauterine growth retardation.
Oligo hydramnios.
Swaddling.
Subluxation is diagnosed in the newborn by means of Ortolani's or Barlow's test, or modifications of these. Mr J. Sharrard FRCS was asked by me to describe Ortolani's test in readily understandable terms. He wrote as follows:

The child is laid on his back with the hip flexed to the right angle and the knees flexed. Starting with the knees together the hips are slowly abducted and if one is dislocated, somewhere in the 90° arc of abduction, the head of the femur slips back into the acetabulum with a visible and palpable jerk. *A mere click in the newborn period is irrelevant*. The diagnosis of dislocation is confirmed by ultrasound.

After 4 or 5 weeks, the most important single sign of subluxation is limited abduction of the hip, with the hips flexed to a right angle. If the subluxation is unilateral, the limitation of abduction is easier to detect, because of the difference between the 2 sides. When the legs are fully extended one should note whether the internal malleoli are exactly opposite each other, for if there is subluxation there is apparent shortening of the limb so that one internal malleolus is higher. When one looks at the soles of the feet the heel on the affected side may be seen to be higher than the other. The child with a missed dislocation of the hip shows, when walking, a characteristic waddling gait (as in muscular dystrophy). If the dislocation is unilateral, there may be toe-walking on the affected side.

Snares in the diagnosis of a dislocated hip
1 Limited abduction of the hip is commonly caused by increased muscle tone, as in cerebral palsy.
    Limited abduction of the hip may be caused by other hip diseases, muscle contracture (p. 56), or congenital shortening or tightness of the adductor muscles.
2 Rarely there is no limitation of abduction of the hip.
3 The hip may dislocate after birth, as it commonly does in cerebral palsy.

Vision

Risk factors
The principal factors which should alert one to the possibility that the baby has a visual defect include the following:
    Nystagmus.
    Familial blindness.

Rubella or other virus infection in early pregnancy.

Severe prematurity.

Mental subnormality.

Cerebral palsy.

Hydrocephalus.

Neonatal ophthalmia.

Modern sophisticated tests for vision in the newborn will not be discussed here.

Inspection of the eye is part of the routine examination of any baby. The newborn may keep his eyes closed, and efforts to force the eyelids open will only make him screw them up more tightly. If one swings the baby around in one's arms, he is likely to open the eyes—at least sufficiently for one to determine whether there is an obvious lens opacity.

A baby with a fixed squint seen at any time from birth should be referred to the ophthalmologist. If a squint is seen or suspected any time after the age of 6 months, the opinion of an ophthalmologist must be obtained. A rare cause of fixed squint or less opacity is a retinoblastoma.

In the case of young infants one can determine whether there is a squint by noting the position of the light reflex on each cornea when a torch is held in front of him. The reflex in each eye should be in the centre of the pupil or at a corresponding point on the 2 corneas.

In testing an older child, one covers one eye with a card while one watches the other eye. When the card is slowly moved away, the eyes should not move if they are straight.

Ability to follow with the eyes, and therefore, to see, is tested with the baby in the supine position by *slowly* moving the shiny handle of a patellar hammer 20–30 cm from the face, and once the baby has seen the object, from the midline to the side or the side to the midline. By 5 or 6 months, near vision is shown by the child reaching out and getting a brick, and when older, a pellet of paper. More distant vision is tested by observing the baby's interest in more distant objects or people, or by deliberately moving the shiny handle of a patellar hammer away from the baby his attention. When in doubt (and always if there is a squint) one consults an ophthalmologist.

The commonest cause of nystagmus in a baby is a defect of vision. Other causes are congenital nystagmus, spasmus nutans and anticonvulsant drugs.

Hearing

Risk factors
The following factors increase the chances that a baby may have a defect of hearing:
Deafness suspected by the parents.
Genetic deafness. Numerous rare syndromes.
Virus infections in pregnancy.
Ototoxic drugs taken in pregnancy or by the child e.g.
    gentamicin, neomycin, streptomycin.
Prematurity, especially if extreme.
    Hyperbilirubinaemia.
Mental subnormality.
Cerebral palsy, especially athetosis.
Meningitis, mumps, mumps vaccine, recurrent otitis
    media.
Sophisticated methods of testing hearing in the newborn will not be discussed here.

In the first 3 months it may be difficult to satisfy oneself that the baby can hear. The sound stimulus is applied 30–45 cm from the ear, on a level with the ear and out of sight of the baby. The sounds are as follows:
PS, PHTH (both for high tones) and OOO for lower
    tones. One must take care not to blow into the ear.
Crinkling paper.
Squeaky toy or small hand bell.
The responses are as follows:
Startle reflex.
A cry.
Quieting if crying.

A blink.

I find that it is sometimes easier to test the baby when he is crying, when one can observe the momentary quieting.

From 3 or 4 months onwards, one tests with the same sounds, at a distance of 30–45 cm from the ear. The child turns his head to sound from 3 or 4 months. One notices in particular the rapidity with which he responds to the sound. The backward child at 6 months may respond only slowly or with difficulty. (At 7 months the normal baby turns his head to sound below the ear and a month later to sound above the ear.)

At 10 months one tests with the sound 90 cm from the ear. When in doubt one seeks the help of an audiologist.

Further reading

Dubowitz L. & Dubowitz V. (1981) Clinics in Developmental Medicine, no. 79. In: *Neurological Assessment of the Newborn Infant*. Spastics International Publication, London.

Illingworth R.S. (1987) *Development of the Infant and Young Child, Normal and Abnormal*, 9th ed. Churchill Livingstone, Edinburgh.

Illingworth R.S. (1988) *Common Symptoms of Disease in Children*, 9th edition. Blackwell Scientific Publications, Oxford.

Index